MG

Notice

The contents of this book or guide are only given as a form of advice and suggestions. If you suffer from any health issues, discuss this book and its contents with your health professional before using it. The author and publisher assume no responsibility or liability for any errors or omissions in the content of this book and do not provide medical advice.

Published by MassoGuide

www.massoguide.com

Copyrighted / Tous droits réservés © 2021 by Maxime Marois.

No part of this publication may be reproduced, distributed, or transmitted in any form or by any means, including photocopying, recording, or other electronic or mechanical methods, without the publisher's prior written permission.

For permission requests, write to the publisher, addressed "Attention: Permission to use," at the address below.

info@massoguide.com

ISBN : 978-1-990512-02-5

First edition - Paper - 2021

In this guide

Introduction

You often hear the word «pressure» when your clients talk about the type of massage they desire. Depth or pressure is indeed one of the key aspects of massage therapy.

When a client consults you and requests a massage with good pressure, you must respond to his needs. This guide is a summary, a collection, and a synthesis of different information and techniques on pressure. They are presented to you in a simple manner to help with your comprehension.

This knowledge aims to help you in your practice by adding a different depth and understanding to your massages.

Happy reading.

Terms glossary

Micromovements:

Very small back and forth movements.

Microrotations:

Very small rotations.

Tensed:

When a muscle fiber is in a contracted state.

Tightness:

When a muscle or the skin is in a state where it feels restrictive and less mobile.

Soreness:

The different sensations you feel when a muscle is touched and there is some discomfort.

Pressure:

Refers to the level of depth that is reached when massaging a muscle. You will generally find the following levels: superficial, medium et deep.

Pain:

Refers to any soreness that has reached the pain threshold.

Health problem:

Any pathology or health issue.

Be advised that this book does not pretend to be a scientific resource but a grouping of different knowledge and techniques to relax tensed muscles.

How to use this

book

Movements

You should follow the instructions on the different illustrations in order to know which area you should massage.

Be sure to take the necessary time to do each movement thoroughly. If you omit parts of the muscle, you will not be relaxing it to its fullest extent.

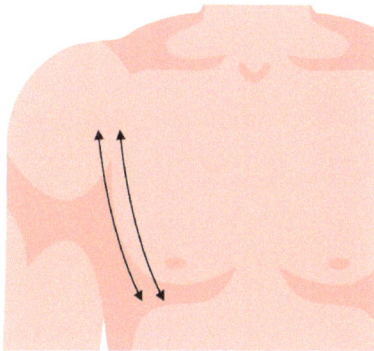

Rotations allow you to relax an area with precision.

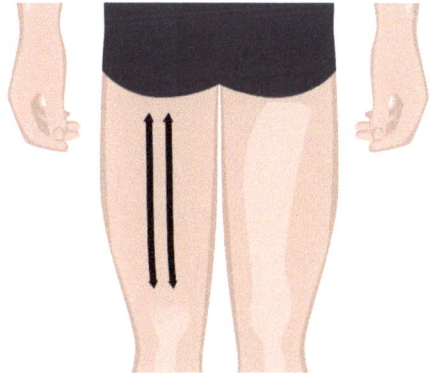

Lines allow you to relax an area or the totality of a muscle.

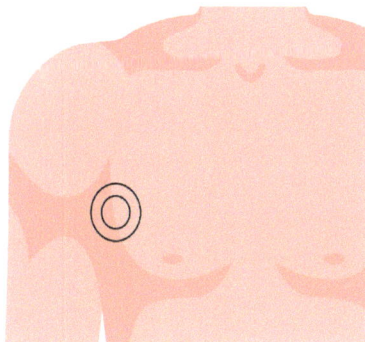

Pressure points allow you to relax slowly the deepest of tensions.

Pressure

To correctly measure the level of soreness felt by your client, be sure to keep communicating about it during the whole duration of the massage. It will help you target the sore spots while not crossing into the unpleasant and painful territory.

Soreness level	Quantity	Description
Almost nothing	0 to 3	The client feels nothing at all or almost nothing.
A little	3 to 5	Relaxes the client, allows to begin the massage slowly, and to explore a client's body to find the tensed areas. It also allows you to massage a very sore area slowly, layer by layer.
Average	5 to 6	Allows you to offer good pressure and to adjust if the area is sore. The ideal level for daily muscle tension.
High	7 to 8	Soreness that is at a high level and approaching the limit.
Very high	8 to 10	Very high level of soreness that the client does not find comfortable. It is also at 10 that the pain level begins, which must not be reached.

Movements and your tools

Excerpt from the book "Techniques for Depth"

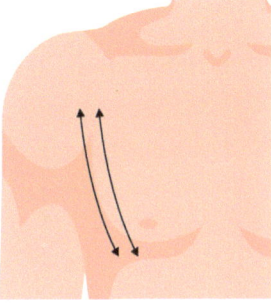

Sliding / Lines

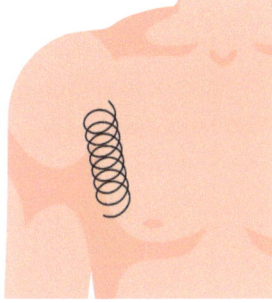

Rotations

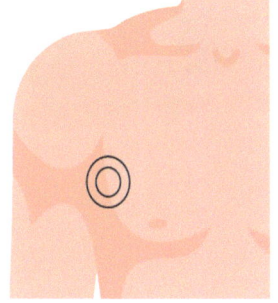

Stationary / Pressure points

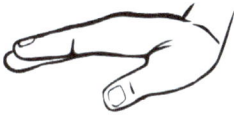

Thumb

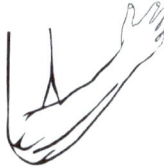

Elbow

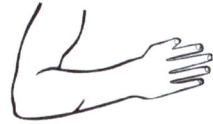

Forearm

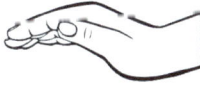

Palm / Effleurage

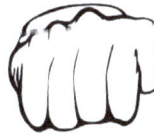

Fist

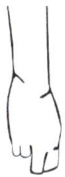

Two fingers

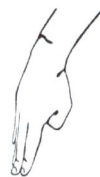

Finger tips

Muscles and their tensions

Levator scapulae

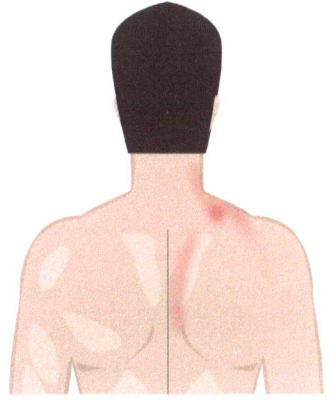

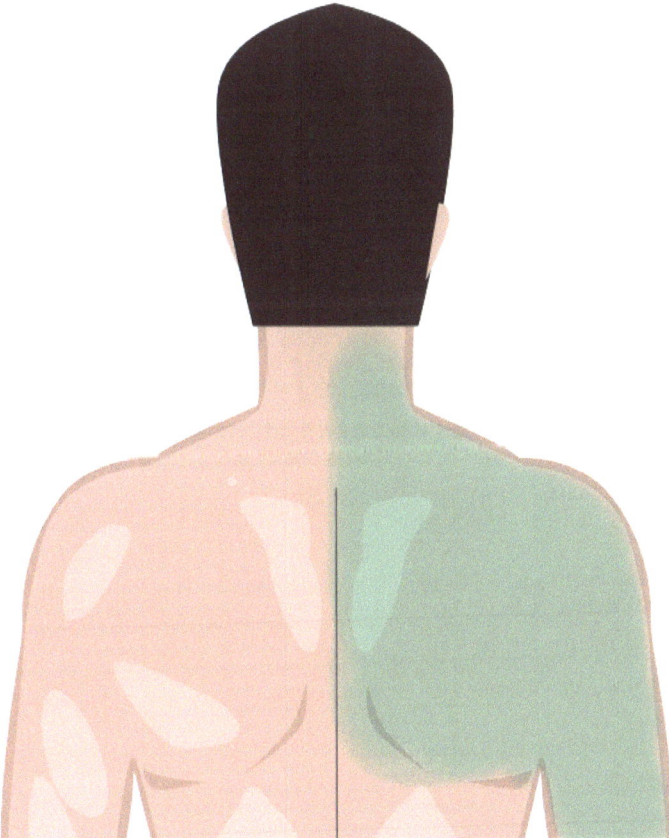

Forearm (continued)

ℹ️ Reason for the tensions: working at the computer, manual work, climbing or other activities of this kind, keeping your hand tightly closed, cleaning with a broom, painting.

Which areas to target :

- Over: Massage between both bones and the thicker area close to the elbow.
- Under: Massage on the side and in the middle. You might notice more tension close to the elbow, which often spreads up to the wrist.
- Elbow: Think about massaging the muscles that are on both sides.

Self-massage tools	Use
Ball	The ball can release the surface tensions and be used for precision work on specific muscles or areas.
Exercises	Stretching can help those who often use their forearms. They will not necessarily efficiently release tensions but can help maintain the area.
Massage gun	The gun is an excellent tool to release tight skin and tensed muscles. However, it will not affect the deepest tensions.

Biceps

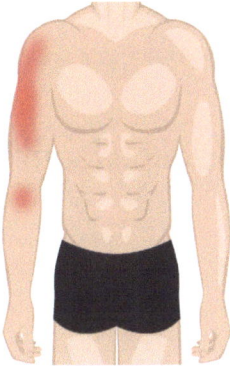

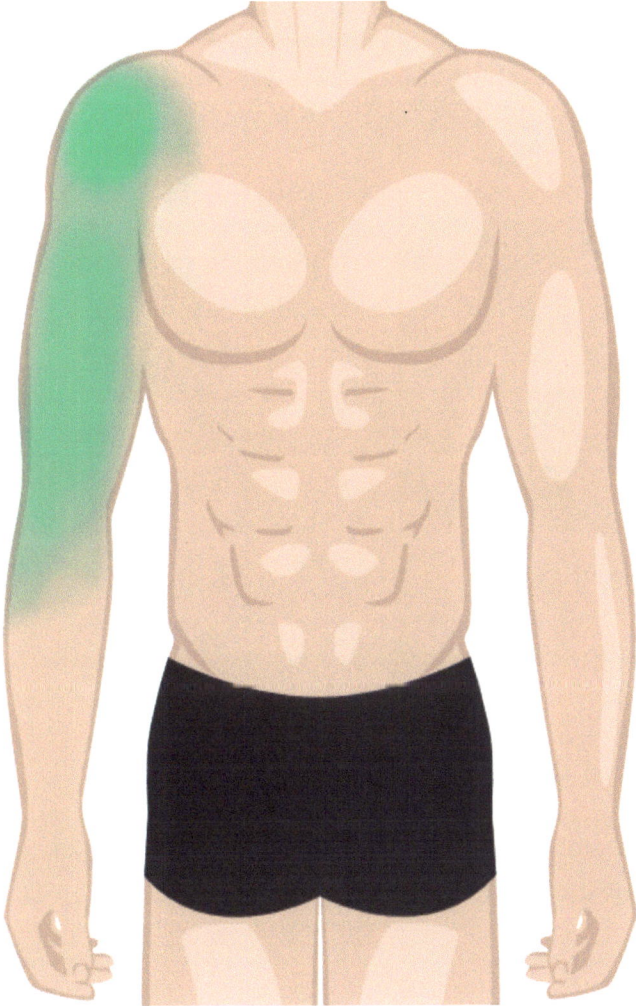

Biceps (continued)

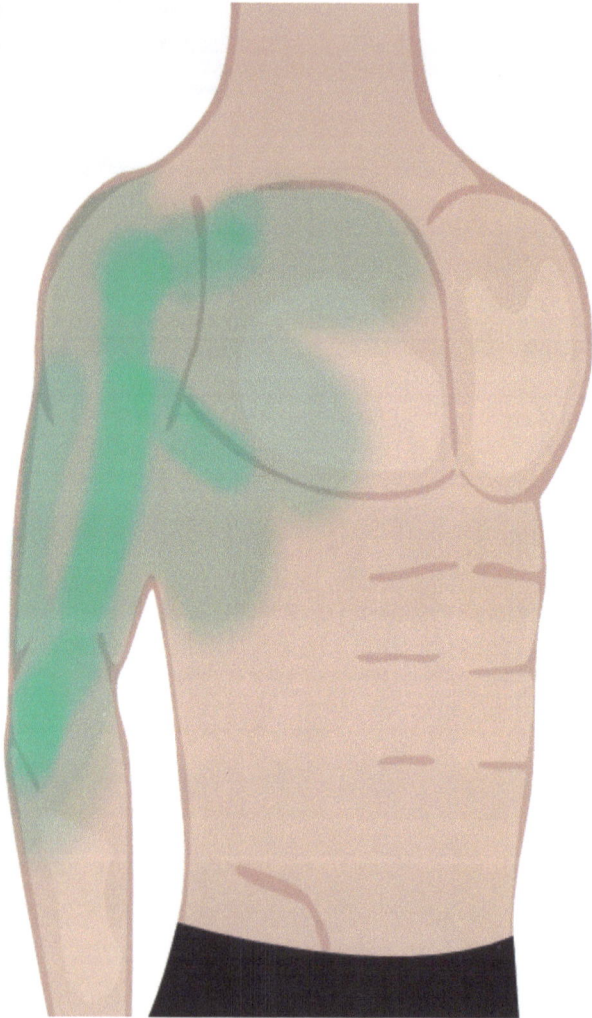

Biceps (continued)

Reason for the tensions :

- Bad posture daily or during training.

Which area to target :

- The muscle on its whole length and the thicker area close to the elbow.

Self-massage tools	Use
Ball	The ball can relax the muscle daily, and it is easy to keep it with you and use it at work.
Exercises	Stretching can help; it will not necessarily release tensions but can help maintain the area.
Massage gun	A gun is an excellent tool to release tensions in this muscle.

Biceps brachialis

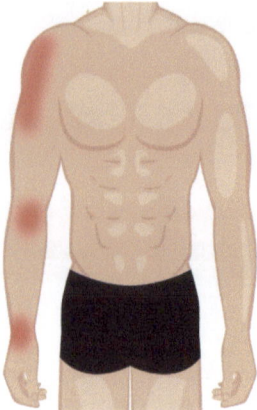

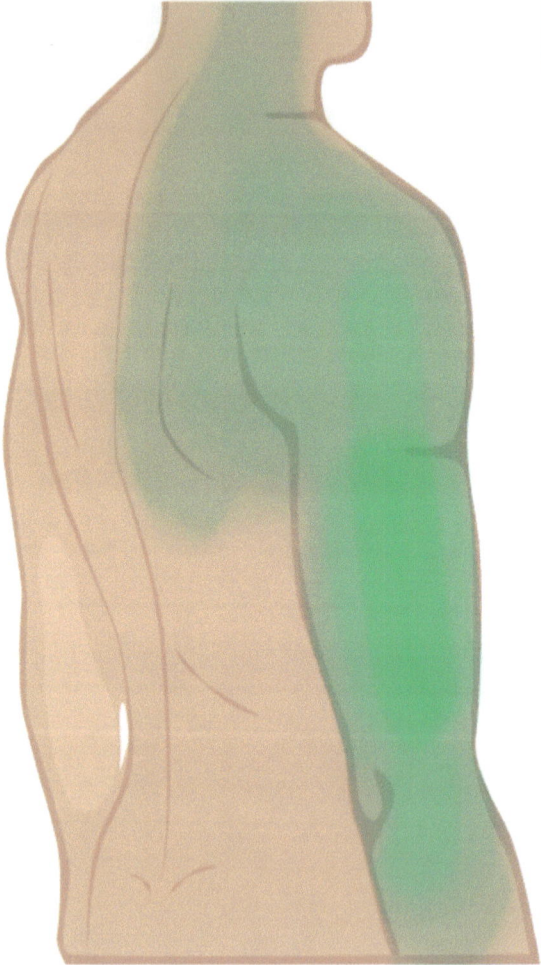

Biceps brachialis (continued)

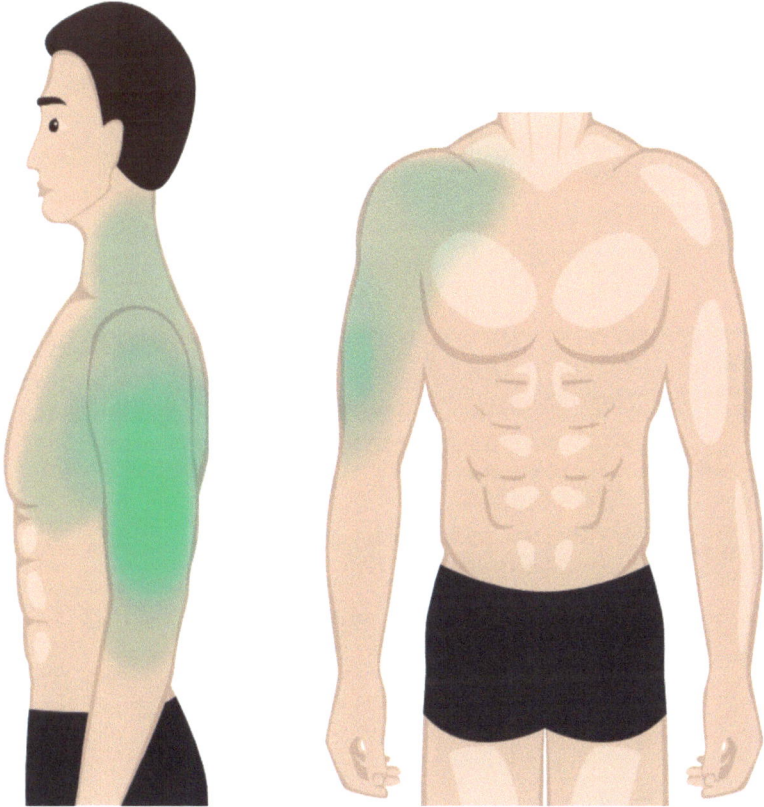

You can open the elbow or move the arm to have access to different parts of the muscle.

Biceps brachialis (continued)

ℹ️ Reason for the tensions: keeping the elbow up in the air, an arm kept tensed or working with the arms in the air.

Which area to target :
- Target the whole muscle as it will be tensed on its whole length.

Self-massage tools	Use
Ball	The ball can reduce most superficial or deep tensions. It can also reduce soreness on the whole arm's length. It can also be easily hidden in a drawer and be used anywhere.
Exercises	Using a stretch is an option for this muscle if it is always tensed. However, it might not release all the tensions that are present.
Massage gun	The gun can be used to release a muscle that seems tight or tensed.

Rotator cuff

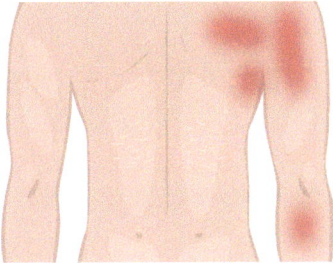

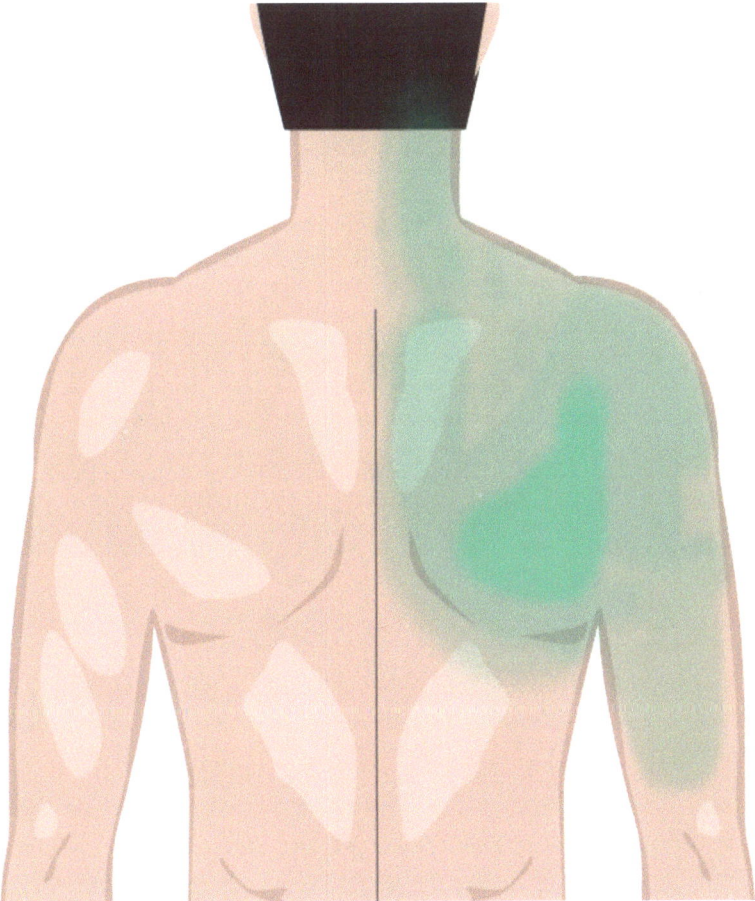

Rotator cuff (continued)

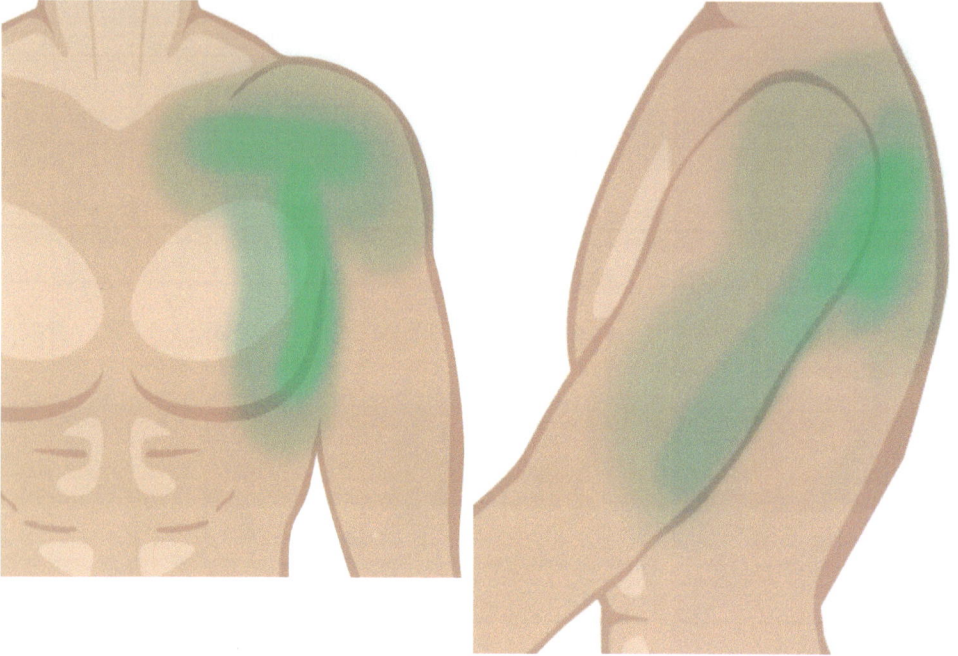

Ribs (continued)

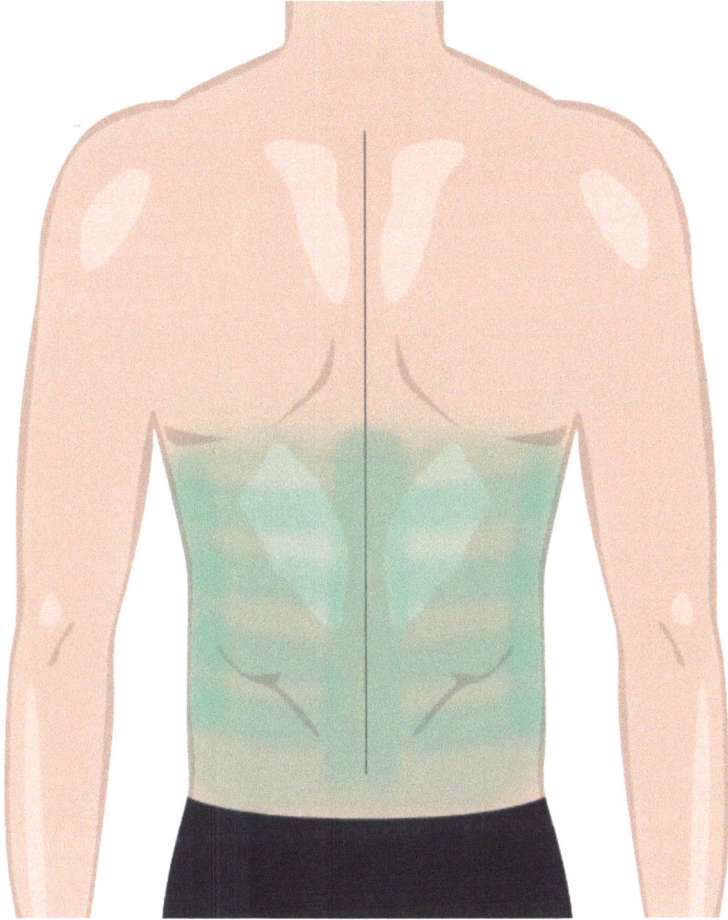

Ribs (continued)

Reason for the tensions:
- leaning on one side
- leaning forward and toward your side

Which area to target :
- Aim for the whole muscle and the individual ribs if they are tensed or sore.

Self-massage tools	Use
Exercises	Stretches will help relax the area and release the tensions.

Deltoid

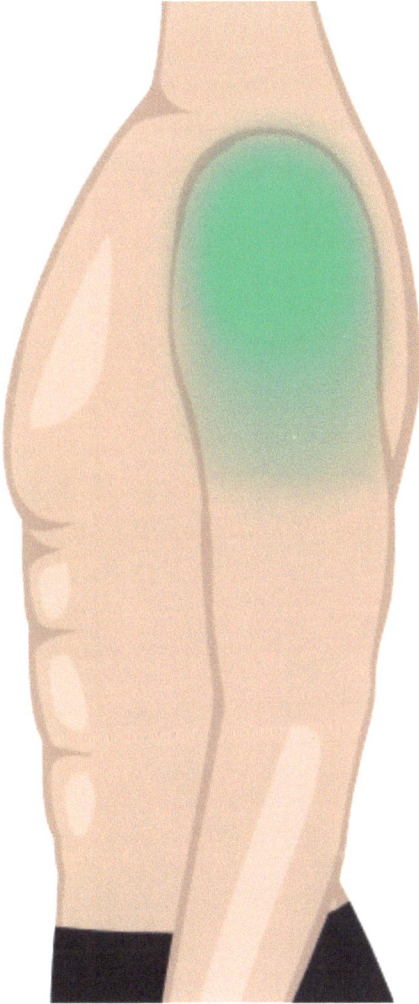

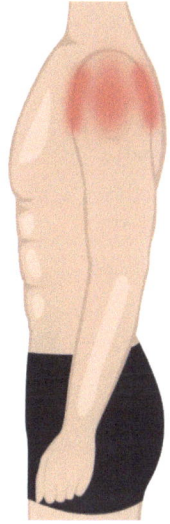

Deltoid (continued)

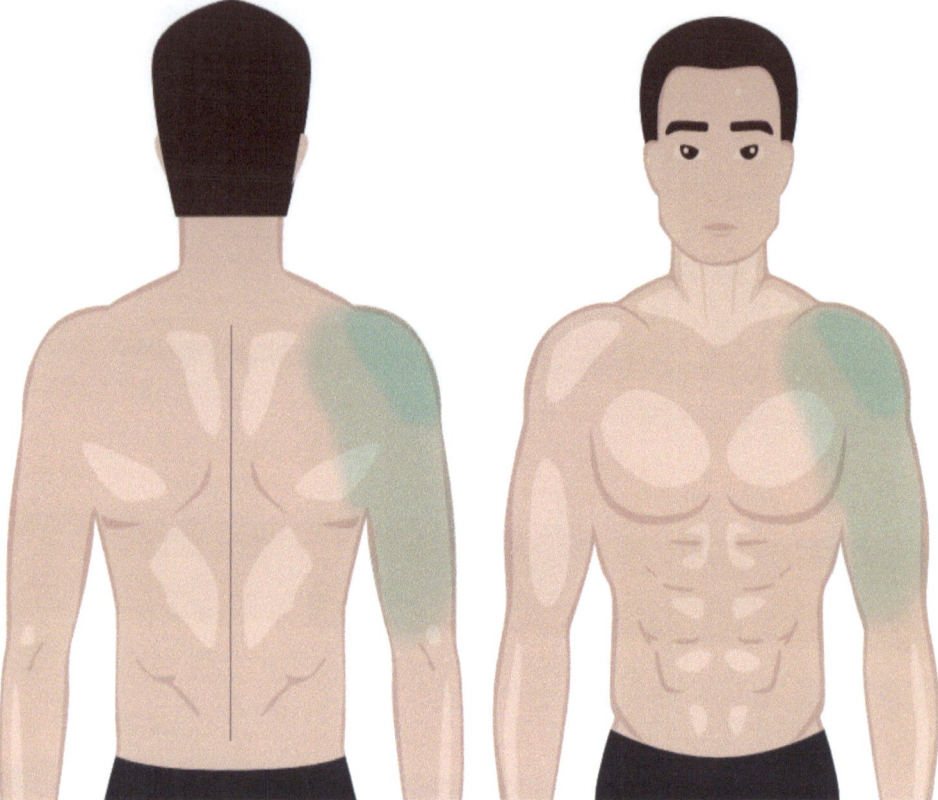

Deltoid (continued)

Reason for the tensions: lousy posture of the arm and/or elbow, leaning forward or working too far away from yourself (such as when using a computer mouse)

Which area to target :
- You can target the whole muscle.

Self-massage tools	Use
Ball	A ball can rapidly relieve soreness in the area and relax it as it is a muscle that's often problematic for office workers; they can also use the ball during their work hours.
Exercises	Stretching can help, but it may retain its soreness.
Massage gun	The gun will release part of the area but will not relax the deepest tensions.

Glutes

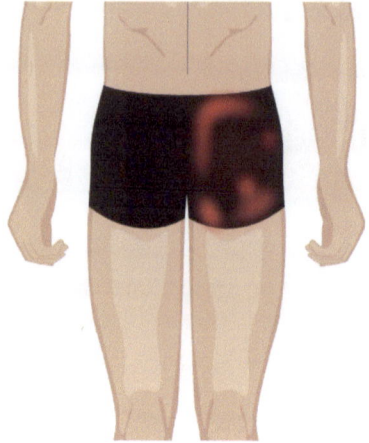

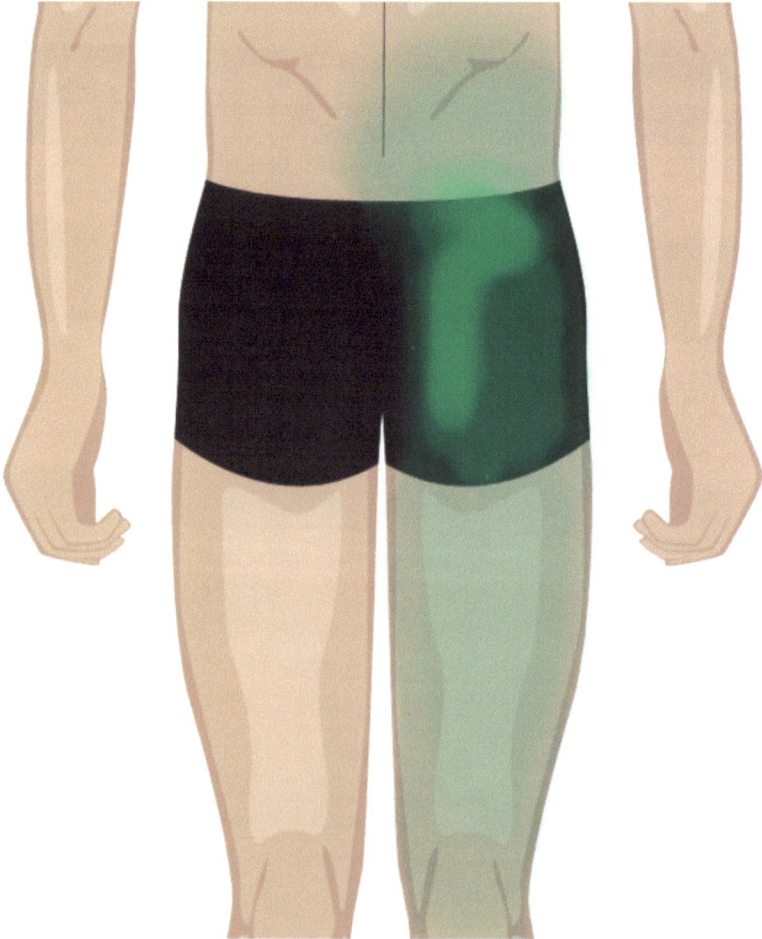

Glutes (continued)

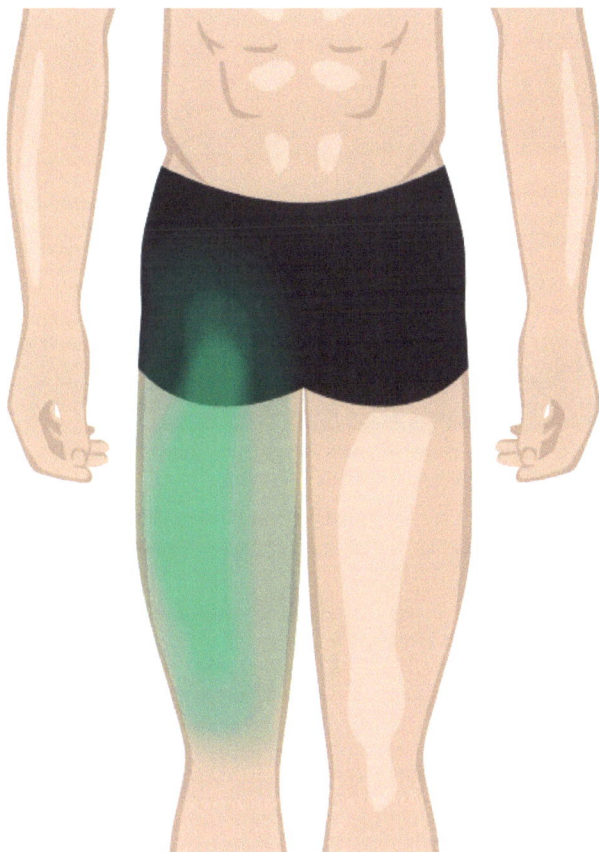

You can rotate the leg during the massage to reach different fibers.

Glutes (continued)

ℹ️ Reason for the tensions: lousy leg or hip posture.

Which area to target :

- Target the extremities as it is where most tensions are.
- Along the muscle to relax it all.
- The muscles that may also impact it.

Self-massage tools	Use
Ball	The ball is generally used for pressure points and to follow the bone along the muscle's insertion points.
Foam roller	The roller can relax the whole muscle, and its edge can massage the edge of the bone behind the glutes. It can also be used for the other muscles surrounding the area.
Exercises	Stretching can relax it and help it to remain relaxed daily, but the deepest fibers might remain tensed.
Massage gun	The massage gun can remove soreness without offering much depth.

Lumbar

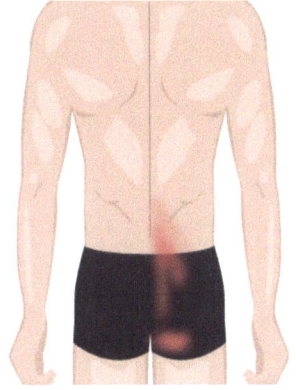

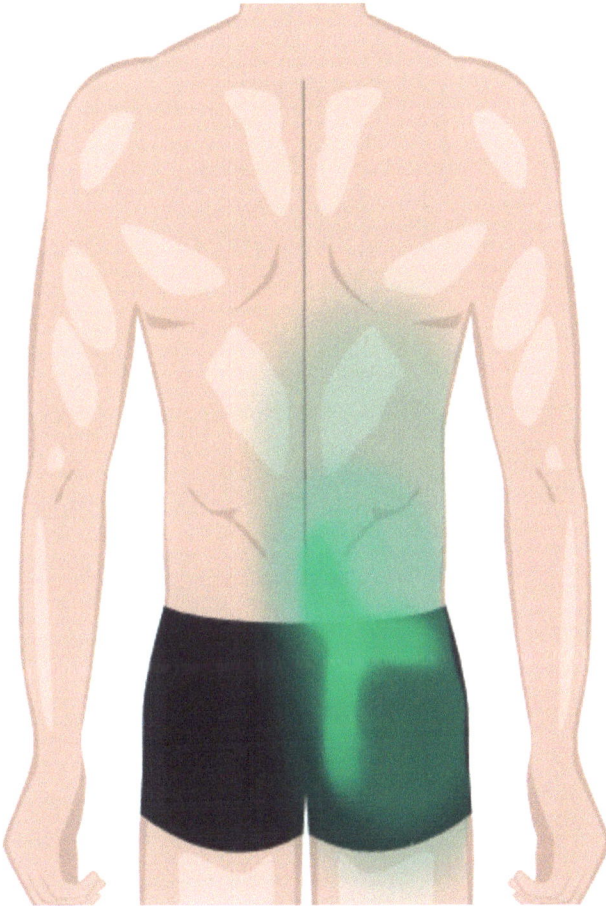

Lumbar (continued)

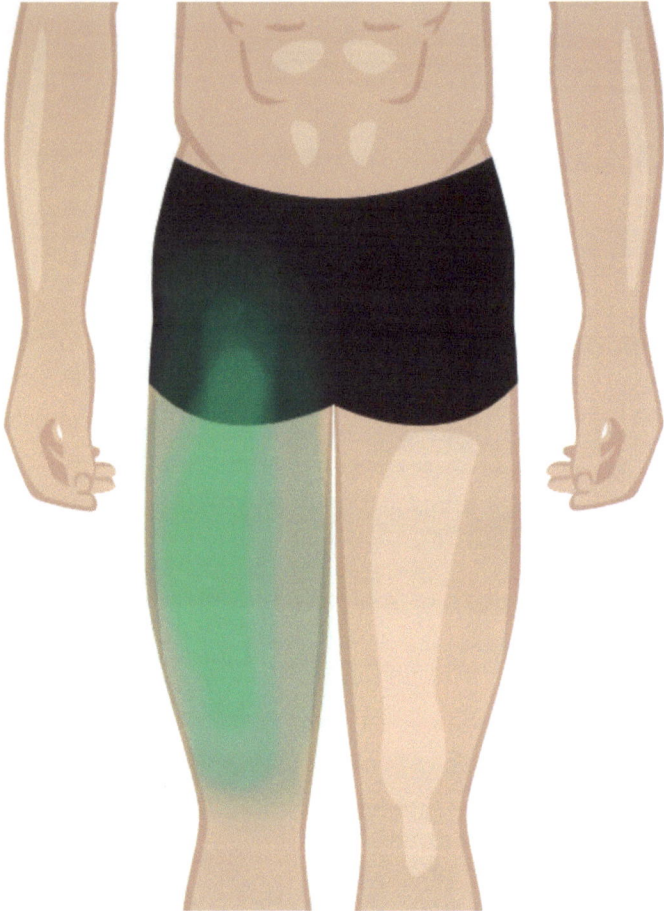

Lumbar (continued)

Reason for the tensions:

- Using the lower back instead of flexing your legs during an effort.
- Sitting with the hips in a poor posture.

Which area to target :

- Massage the lower back muscles.
- Along the spine in this area.
- The glutes' insertion points.

Self-massage tools	Use
Exercises	You can use other tools, but the stretch allows a precise relaxing of the tensions.

Hand

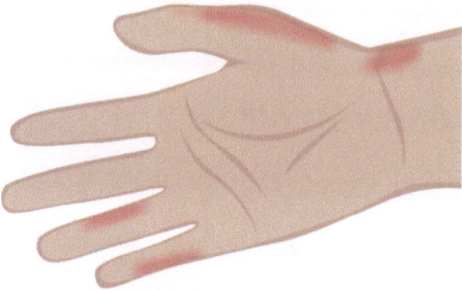

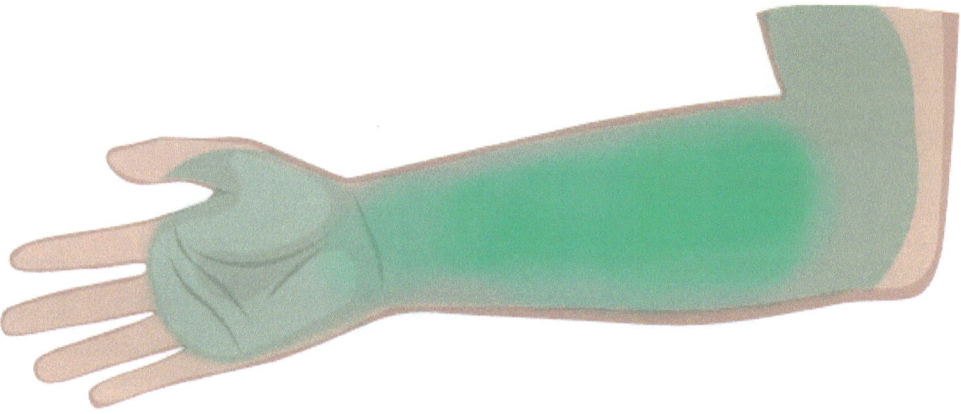

Hand (continued)

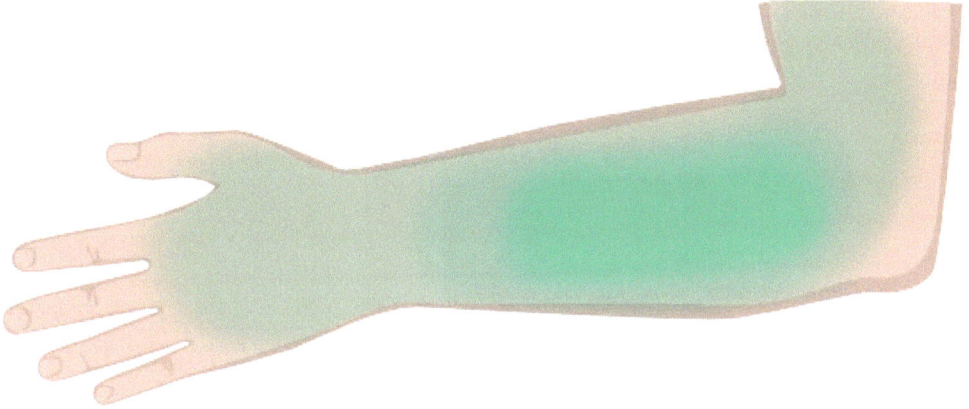

Reason for the tensions:

- If the hand is often used, it will develop tensions.

Which area to target :
- Thumb: You can relax tensions between the thumb and the index finger.

- Palm: Relax the different spaces between each bone. You can also mobilize different parts of the hand to help them relax.

Self-massage tools	Use
Ball	The ball is handy for quick release, and it can be easily carried and used at work.
Exercises	You can stretch the hands and possibly of the forearms.
Massage gun	The gun will rapidly relax the hand, but it will not relieve the deepest tensions, such as the ones in the thumb.

Calf

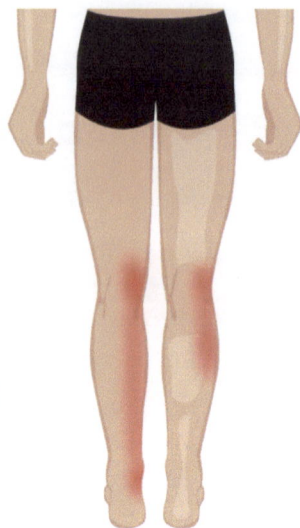

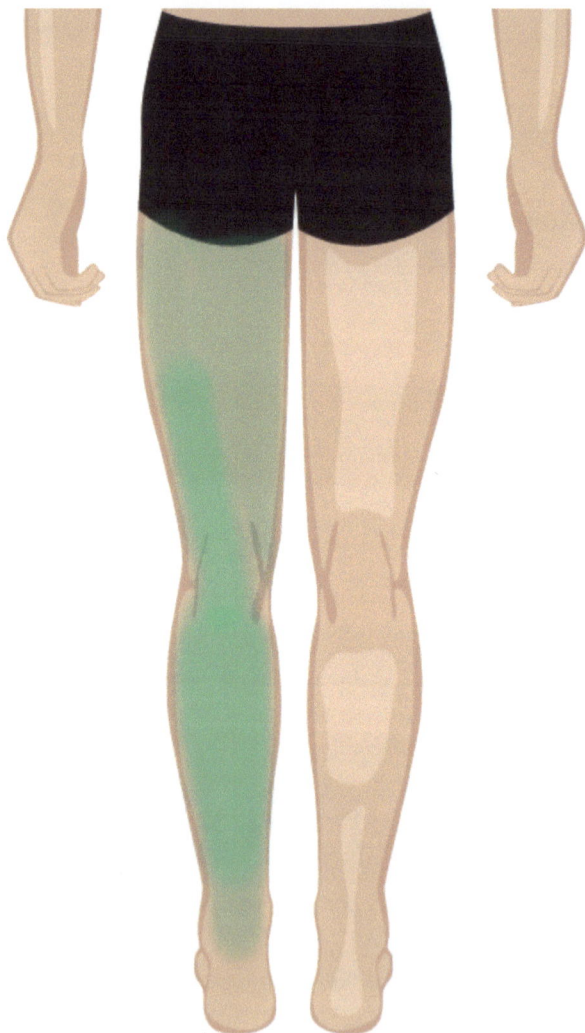

Calf (continued)

Reason for the tensions:

- Soreness after training, sport tensions, bad postures.
- External calf: External rotation of the leg.

Which area to target :

- Do not forget the extremities as they can often be sore.
- You will find tensions along the whole length of the muscle.
- External calf
- Internal calf

Self-massage tools	Use
Ball	The ball can be used, but it can be more challenging in some cases.
Foam roller	The roller can be used, but it can also be difficult.
Exercises	You can release some tensions by stretching the muscle.
Massage gun	The gun can loosen some of the most superficial tensions. The vibration will also help relax tho whole muscle.
Knee	You can self-massage some areas with the knee by placing the muscle onto it with the legs crossed.

Neck

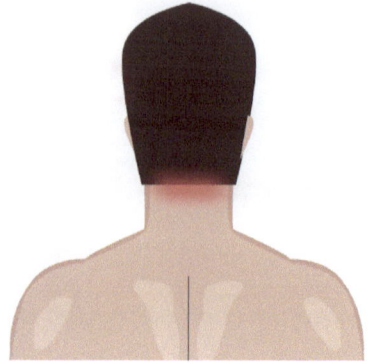

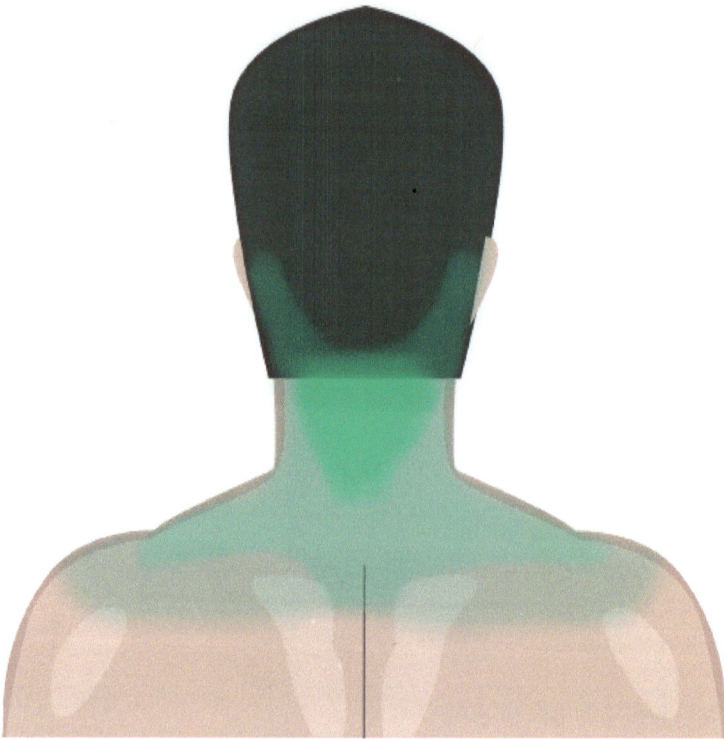

Variation: You could find that massaging those areas is easier when your client is laying on his/her back.

Neck (continued)

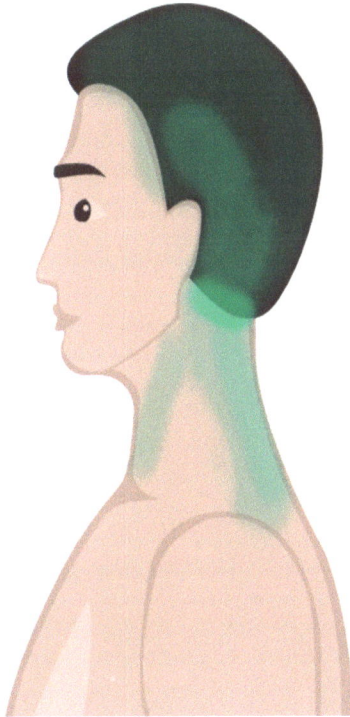

You can move the head in multiples ways to have better access to different muscles.

Variations:

- Turning it on the side.
- Bringing it closer to the shoulder.
- Bringing it further from the shoulder.
- Doing a mix of the previous.

Neck (continued)

ℹ️ Reason for the tensions: Bad postures daily or serious effort.

Which area to target :

- Splenius muscles

- Semispinalis muscles

- Rectus capitis posterior major

- Rectus capitis posterior minor

- Obliquus capitis superior

- Obliquus capitis inferior

- Head

- Trapezius

- Levator scapulae

- Scalene muscle

Self-massage tools	Use
Ball	A ball, placed under a towel, can give good access to this area and to the sore and deep tensions.
Foam roller	The roller can help replicate some of what the ball can do, but it remains limited and is not the best for this job.
Exercises	Stretching can rapidly relax tensions and help in keeping this area relaxed over time.
Massage gun	The gun can relax those areas; however, it can be problematic if used close to the occipital region.
Hand	Your clients can also use their hands and fingers to relax the area.

Foot

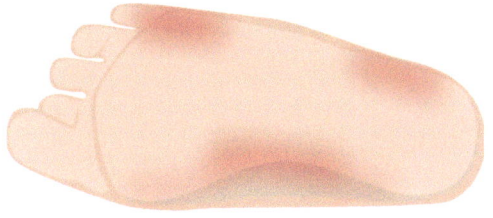

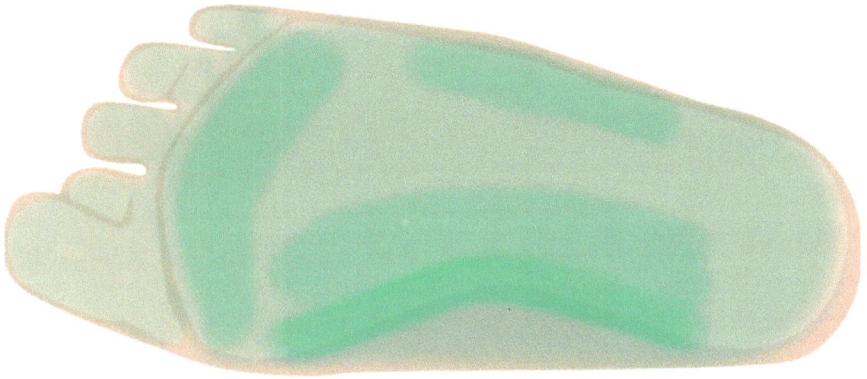

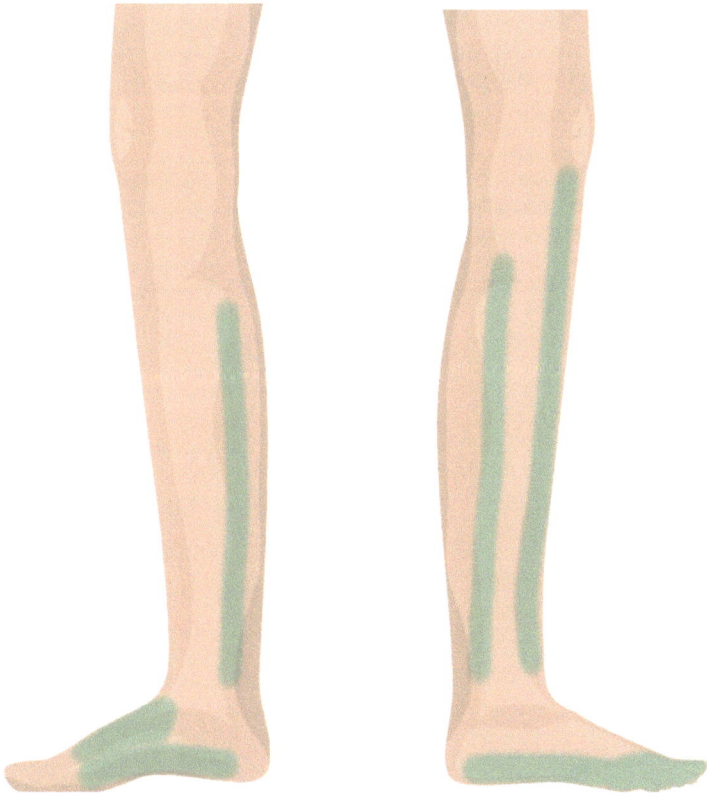

44

Foot (continued)

ⓘ Reason for the tensions: bad posture, lack of mobility, accumulation, lack of mobility.

Which area to target :

- Arch: relax the whole area.

- Heel: You can slowly mobilize the heel with your hand using a light grip.

- The thicker area below the toes: massage all over the area.

- Between the bones: relax the muscles that are between the bones of the foot. You can massage them with the thumb or mobilize them.

Self-massage tools	Use
Ball	You can easily massage the foot with a ball.
Mobilizing	You can mobilize the client's foot, or he can do that himself by moving each bone in different directions carefully. It creates a small massage and allows you to move the muscles in different directions, speeds and angles.
Massage gun	The gun can relax the feet's muscles, but it is not a complete solution.

Quads

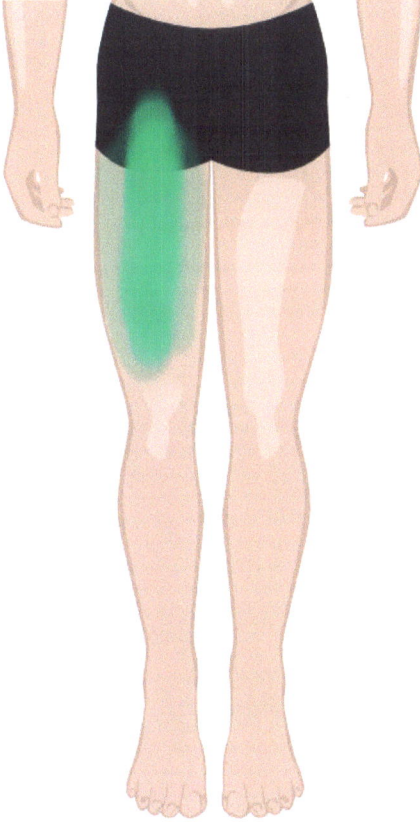
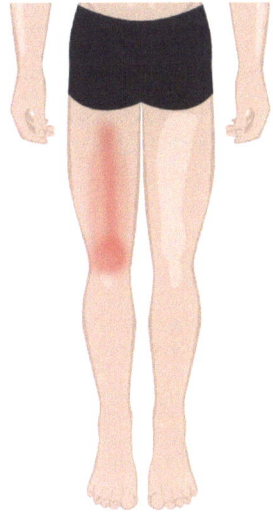

Quads (continued)

i Reason for the tensions: Bad posture, strenuous effort, lack of maintenance of the muscles over time.

Which area to target :

- The whole muscle.

- You can find more tensions closer to the extremities.

Self-massage tools	Use
Ball	The ball can relax a muscle that's too sore.
Foam roller	The roller allows you to relax the whole muscle and to vary the depth/soreness to maximize your effort.
Exercises	Stretching allow you to isolate the muscle to relax easily.
Massage gun	The gun can relax the most superficial tensions.

Quads (external)

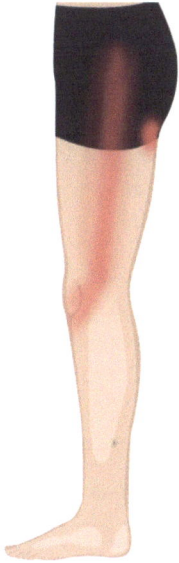

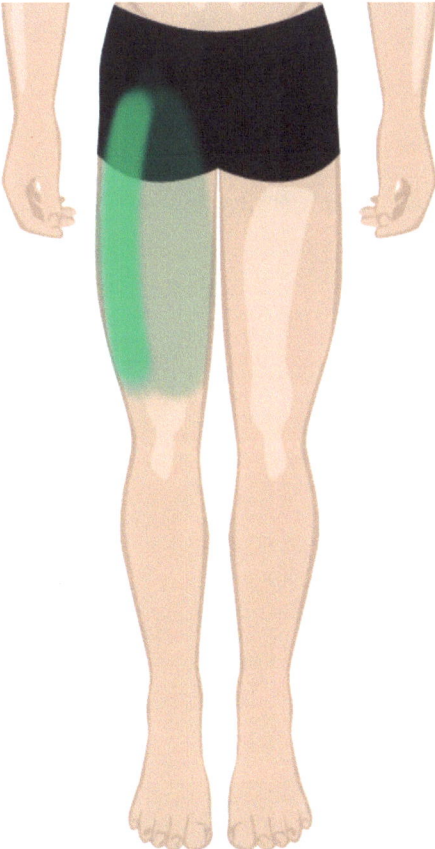

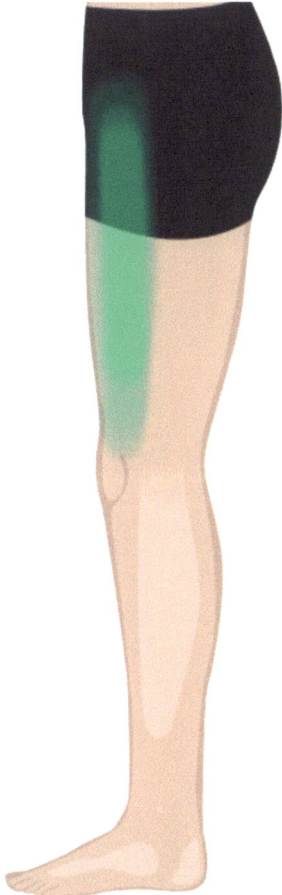

Quads (external) (continued)

ℹ️ Reason for the tensions: Keeping your legs open repeatedly when sitting or standing, keeping
the legs crossed, a bad posture of the legs/knees while cycling.

Which area to target :

- Extremities

- The whole muscle

Self-massage tools	Use
Ball	The ball can relax or relieve soreness on parts of the area.
Foam roller	The roller allows you to massage the deepest tensions.
Exercises	Stretching can release the sorest tensions for some time.
Massage gun	The gun can relax the superficial tensions.

Rhomboid

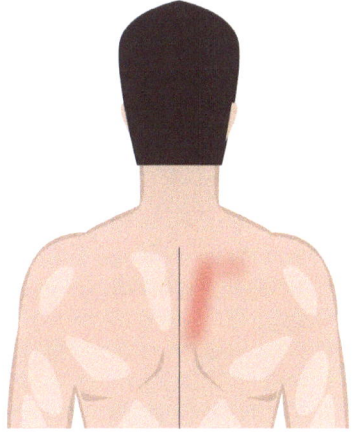

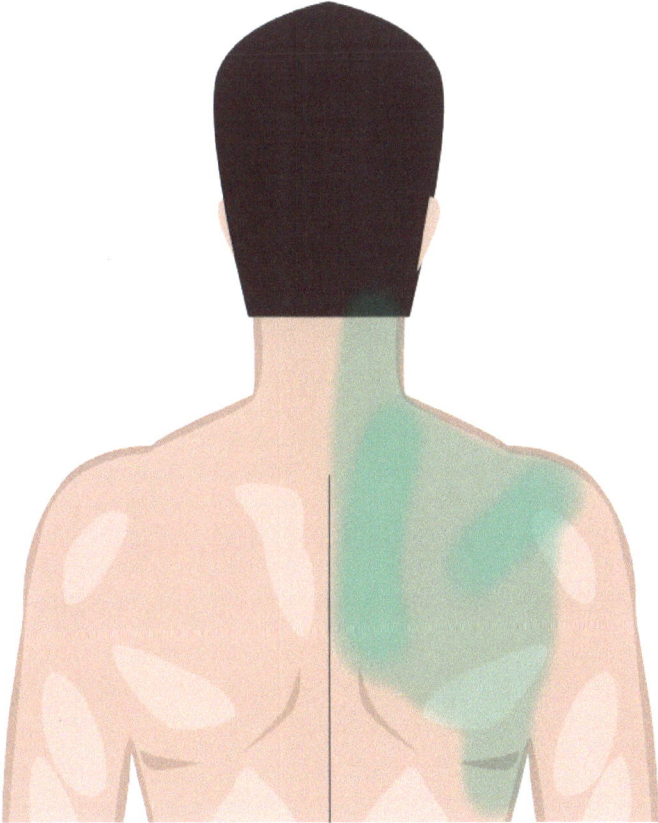

Rhomboid (continued)

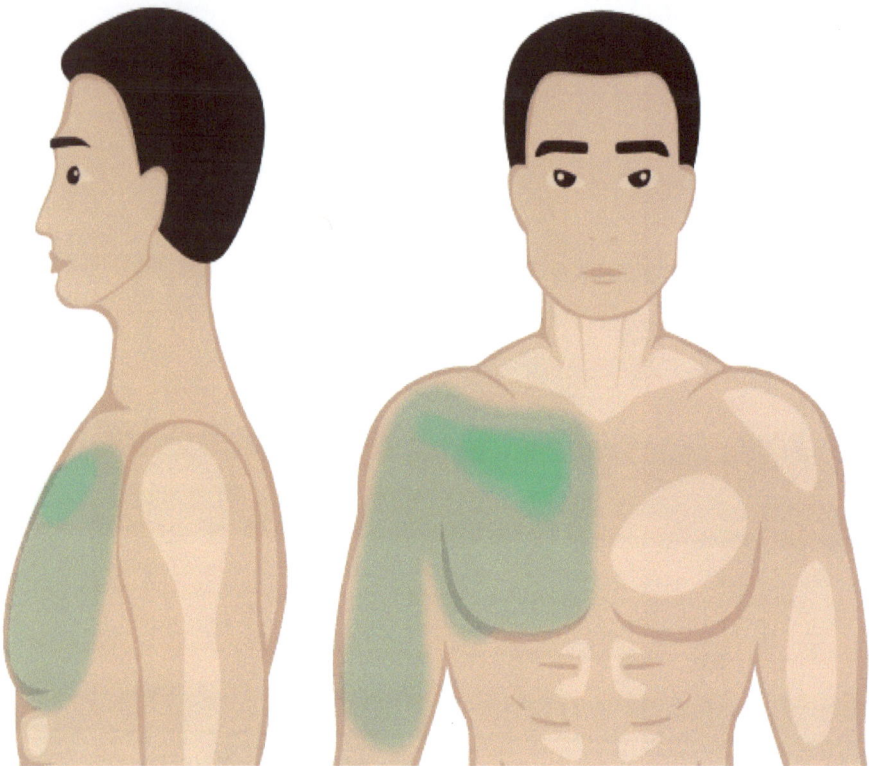

Rhomboid (continued)

Reason for the tensions:

- bad shoulder posture: too forward, leaning on it during long periods

- bad arm posture

Which area to target :

- Between the spine and the scapulae.

- All along its insertions on the scapulae.

Self-massage tools	Use
Ball	The ball is often used for a pressure point on the muscle. It is also possible to do micromovements to relax the muscle.
Foam roller	Perpendicularly placed against the muscle, it can relax it by doing a pressure points or micromovements.
Exercises	Stretch the muscles that are connected to the rhomboid.
Massage gun	The gun can temporarily ease soreness in the area.

Spinalis

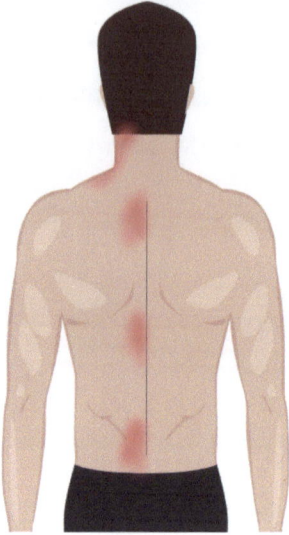

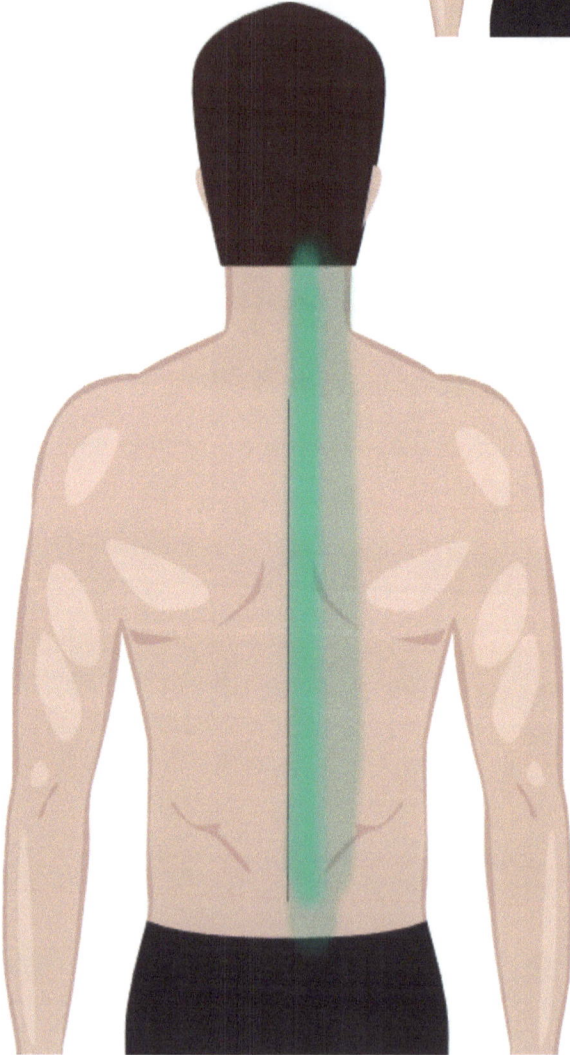

Spinalis (continued)

Reason for the tensions: efforts and/or bad postures.

Which area to target :

- The muscle directly.

- The sorest area is generally in the middle of the back, at the same height as the lowest part of the scapulae.

- You can also look close to the ribs to find tensed muscles.

Self-massage tools	Use
Ball	You can use one or two balls to make pressure points or to slide.
Foam roller	The roller offers the best depth and the ability to massage the muscle thoroughly and quickly.
Exercises	Stretching alleviates the most annoying tensions.
Massage gun	The gun can help to relax the area.

Subclavius

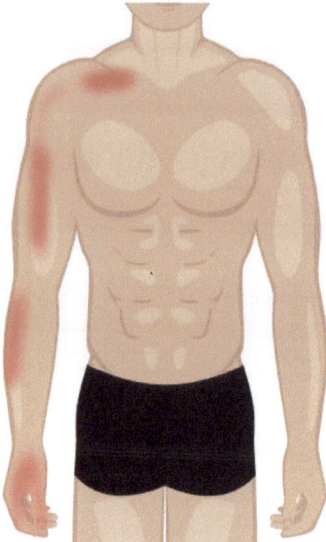

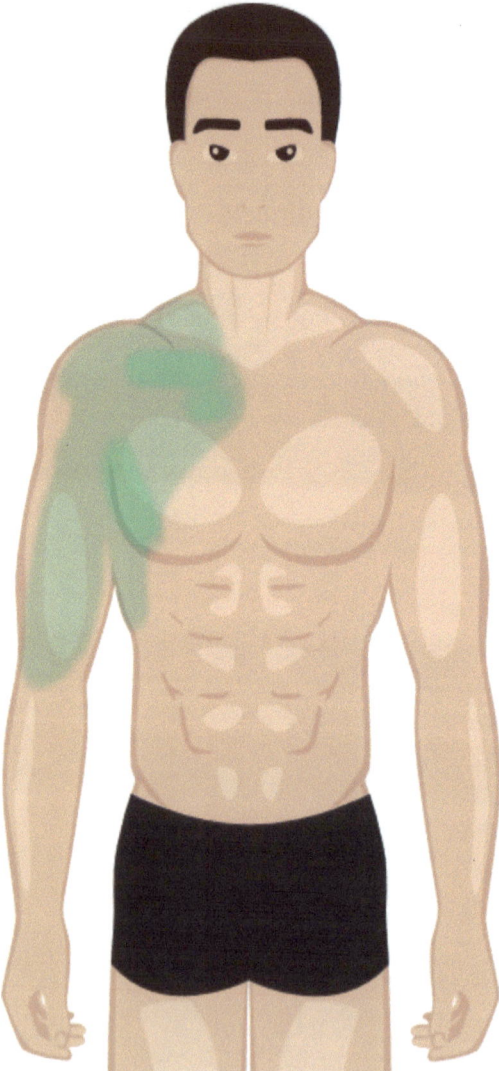

Subclavius (continued)

Reason for the tensions: Leaning forward and/or when the arm is too forward to work further from you.

Which area to target :

- Follow the muscle on its whole length as it is tiny and therefore requires precision.

Self-massage tools	Use
Ball	You can use the ball to massage this area and the small pectorals muscles.
Massage gun	The gun can release the whole area without precisely targeting this muscle.

Subscapularis

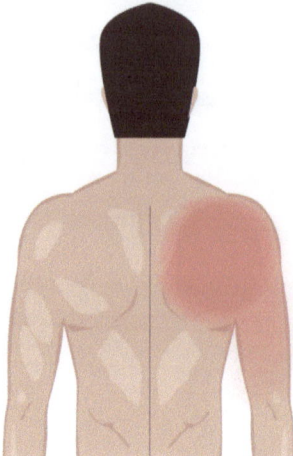

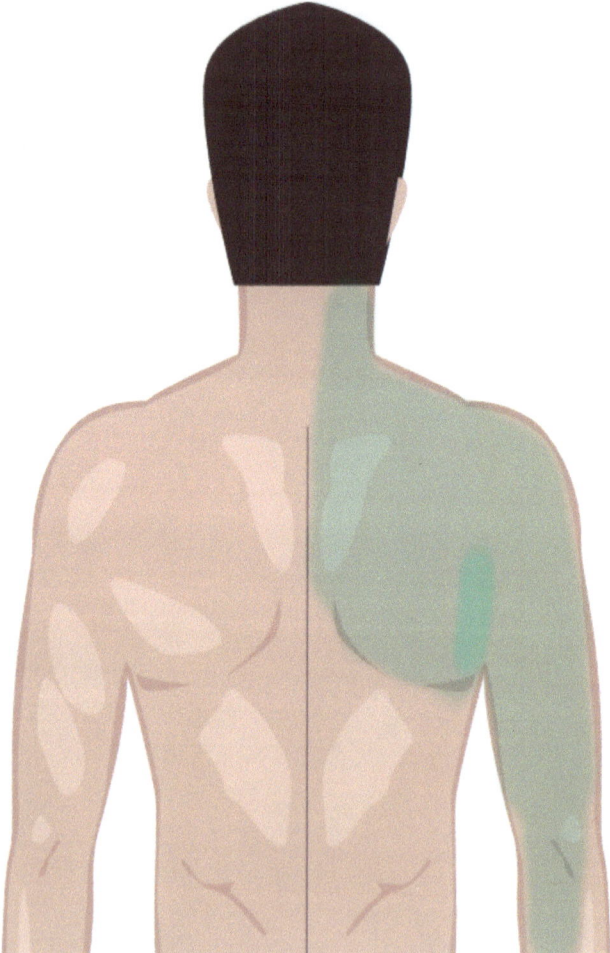

Subscapularis (continued)

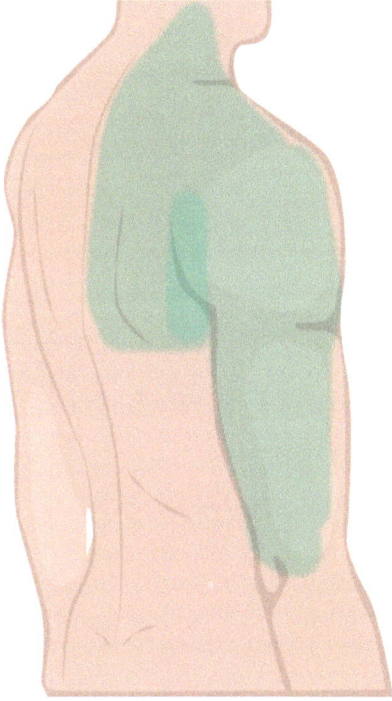

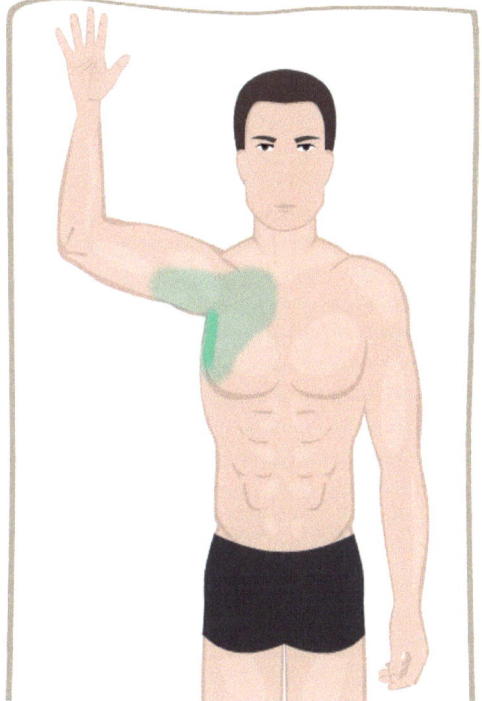

Variation: You can open the elbow or move the arm to have access to different parts of the muscle.

Subscapularis (continued)

ℹ️ Reason for the tensions: tricep extension when leaning, leaning on the shoulder.

Which area to target :

- The area that you can easily access by the armpit.

Self-massage tools	Use
Fingers	You can use your finger to massage the muscle directly.
Exercises	Using a stretch is an option if the muscle is always tensed, but it might not release the tensions.
Massage gun	Massage the area by accessing it via the armpit.

Tensor fasciae latae (TFL)

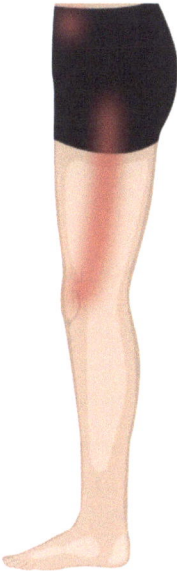

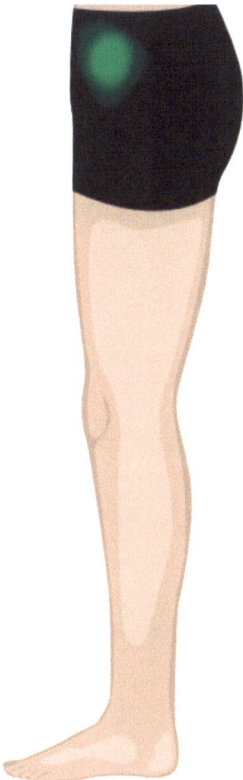

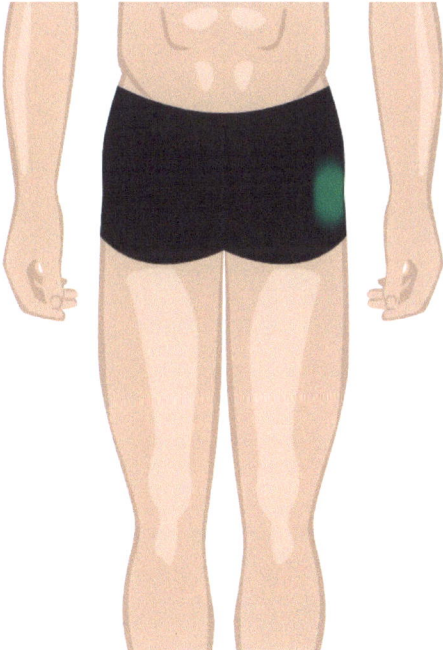

Tensor fasciae latae (TFL) (continued)

ⓘ Reason for the tensions: keeping your legs open repeatedly (sitting or standing), bad posture when you do squats, crossing the legs.

Which area to target :

- The muscle itself, not the iliotibial band (IT band).

Self-massage tools	Use
Ball	You can make a static pressure point to relax the muscle, but it can be pretty sore.
Exercises	You can stretch the muscle to relax some of the tensions.
Massage gun	Use the gun statically to relax the muscle.

Tibialis anterior

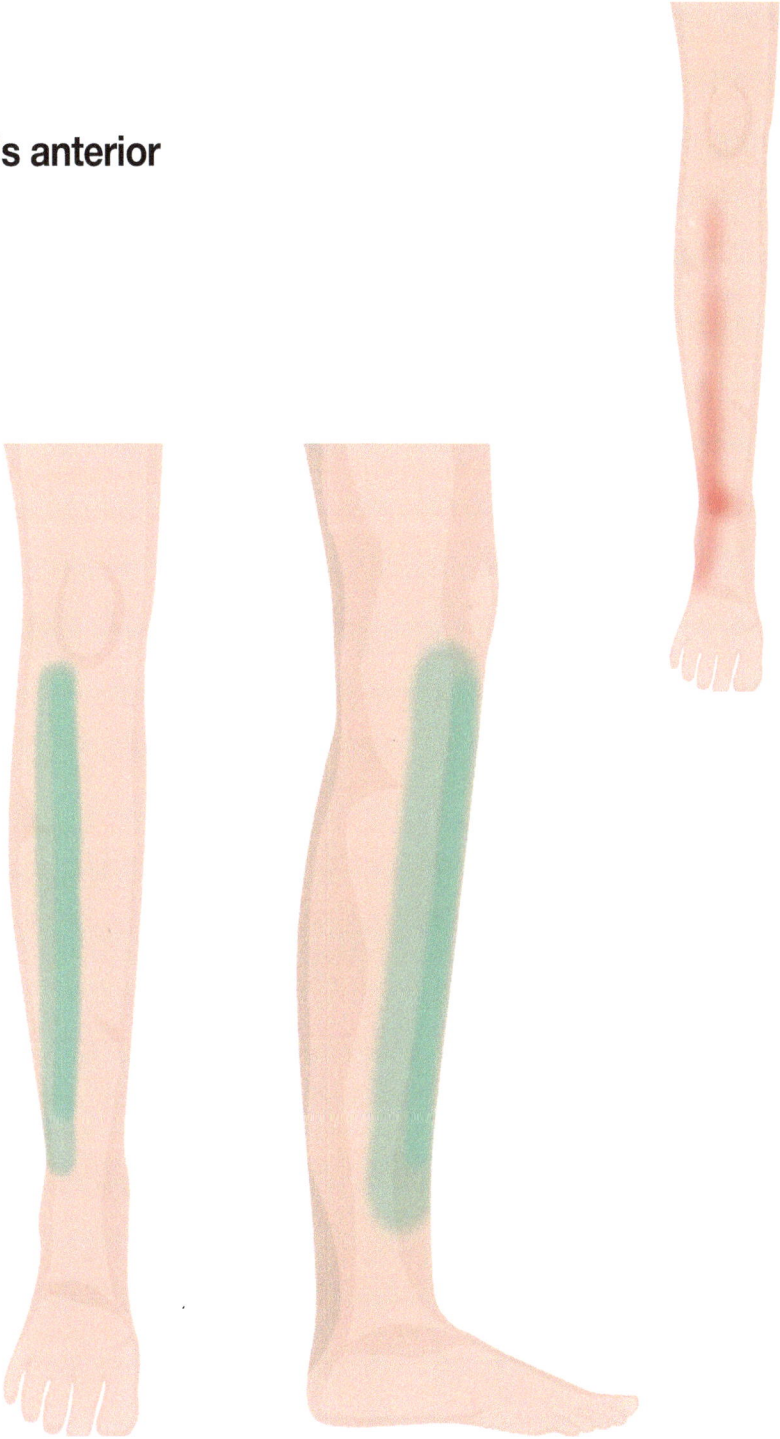

Tibialis anterior (continued)

ℹ Reason for the tensions: Bad posture when sitting, physical activity.

Which area to target :

- The whole muscle.

Self-massage tools	Use
Ball	The ball can relieve soreness and work in depth.
Massage gun	The gun is helpful for the client and for the therapist when trying to release the area.

Trapezius (transverse)

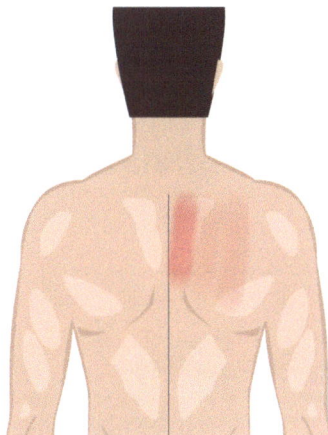

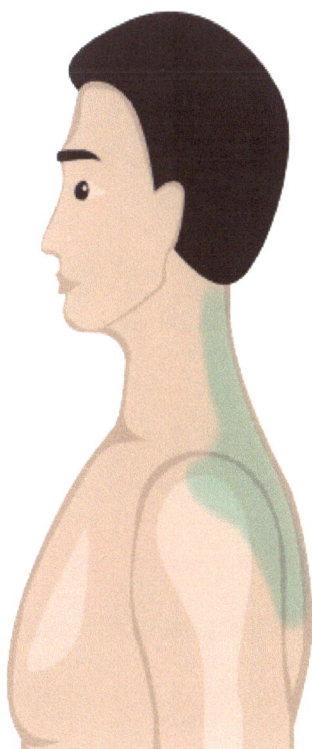

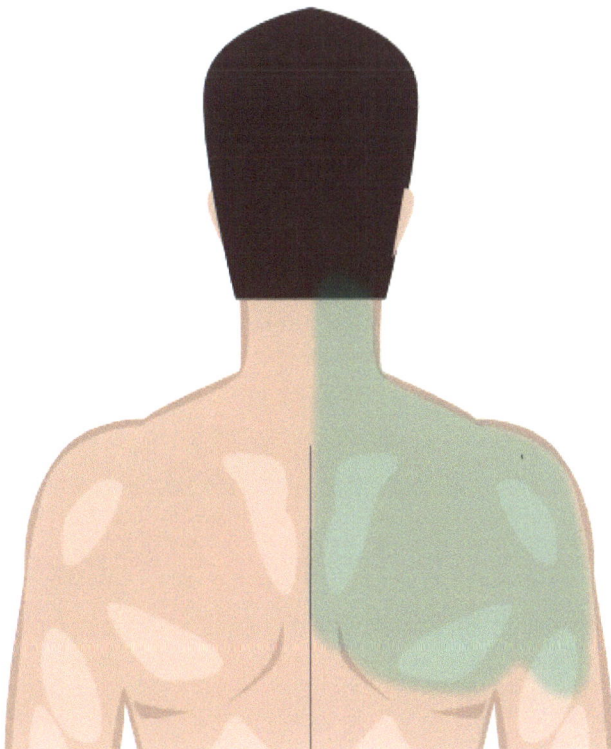

Trapezius (transverse) (continued)

ℹ Reason for the tensions: lousy shoulder or back posture.

Which area to target :

- The whole muscle: on the rhomboid, the scapulae, and behind the shoulder.

Self-massage tools	Use
Ball	It can be challenging to massage this muscle with a ball.
Foam roller	You can use the roller on some parts of the muscle.
Massage gun	The gun is hard to use alone without assistance and might not release all tensions.

Trapezius (superior)

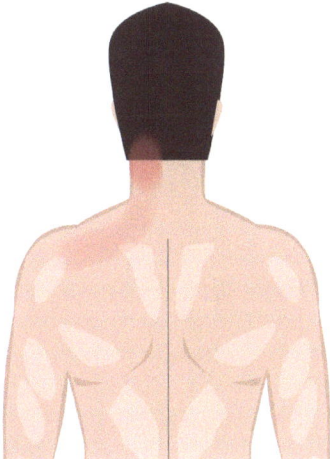

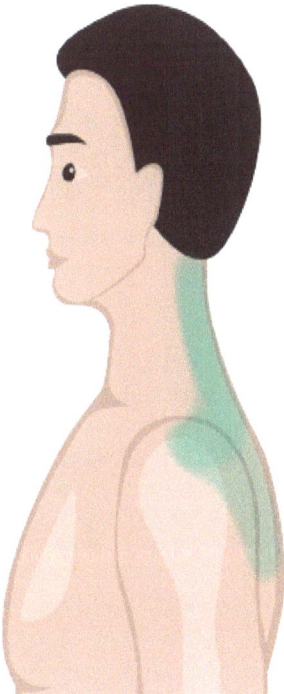

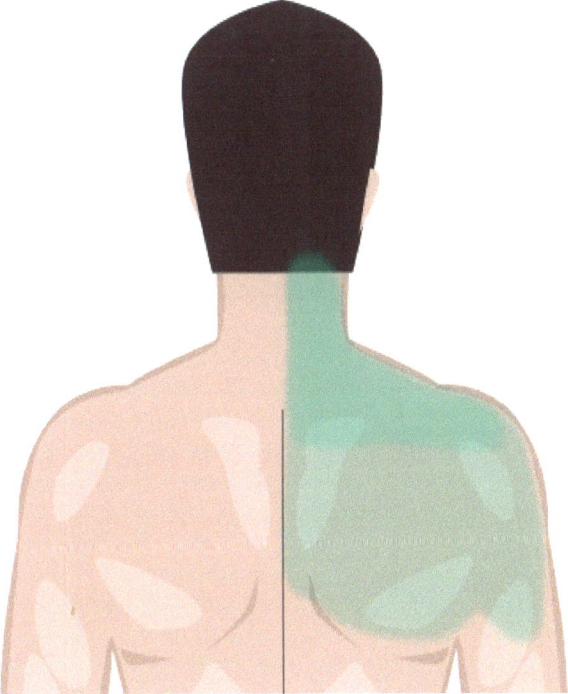

Trapezius (superior) (continued)

ℹ Reason for the tensions: lousy posture or strenuous efforts with the arm, the head, the shoulder, or the back.

Which area to target :

- Follow the muscle on its whole length as it is not always uniformly tensed.

- Look at the pectoralis muscles and/or the length of the arm to see if the areas are tensed.

Self-massage tools	Use
Exercises	Stretching can help relax the area but will need to include other muscles.
Massage gun	The gun can release a lot of the most superficial tensions.

Pectoralis major

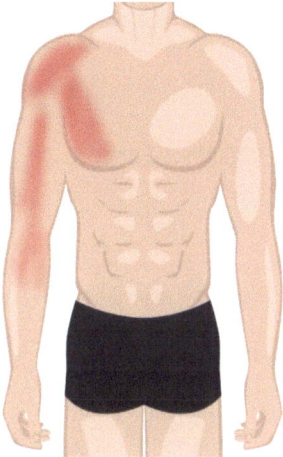

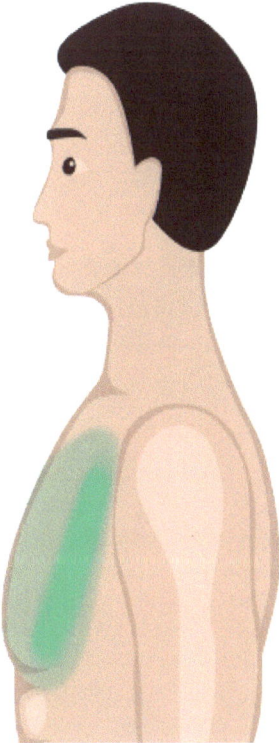

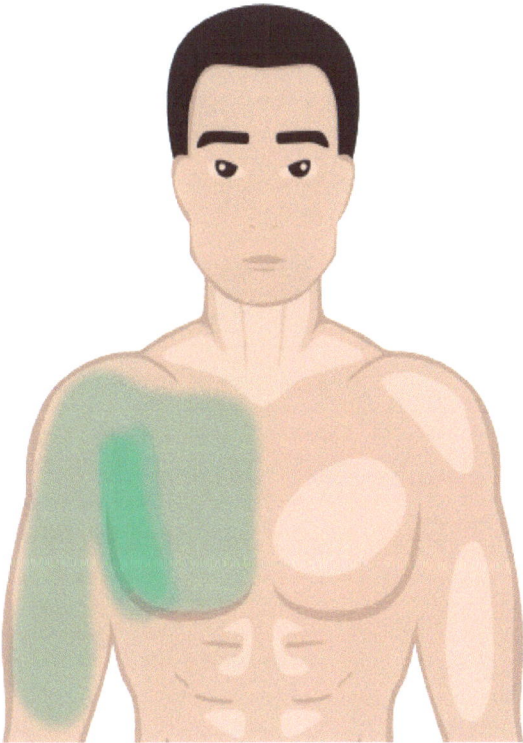

Pectoralis major (continued)

ℹ Reason for the tensions: Bad upper body posture

Which area to target :

- Along the thicker external part: you can access it by massaging along the armpit.

- Close to the head of the humerus bone: you will often find tensions in this area and especially if the muscle is contracted for long periods.

- *Warning: it is possible that your clients feel electric shocks or tingling sensations in the hand when you massage this area. Adjust the pressure and/or alternate by massaging other muscle parts before coming back on this area. It happens because many important nerves are below this area.

Self-massage tools	Use
Ball	The ball will easily relax the muscle and release tensions.
Exercises	Stretching can be helpful if it seems very tense and cannot be relaxed by self-massage or even during the massage.
Massage gun	You can use the gun when the ball, correctly and sufficiently used, cannot release all the tensions in the area.

Pectoralis minor

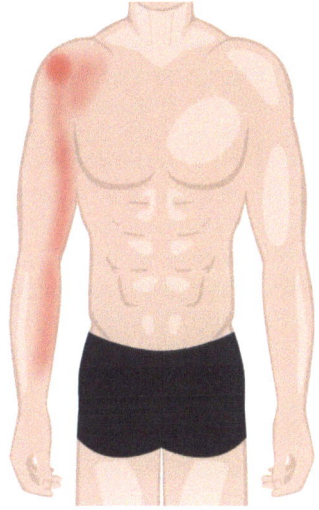

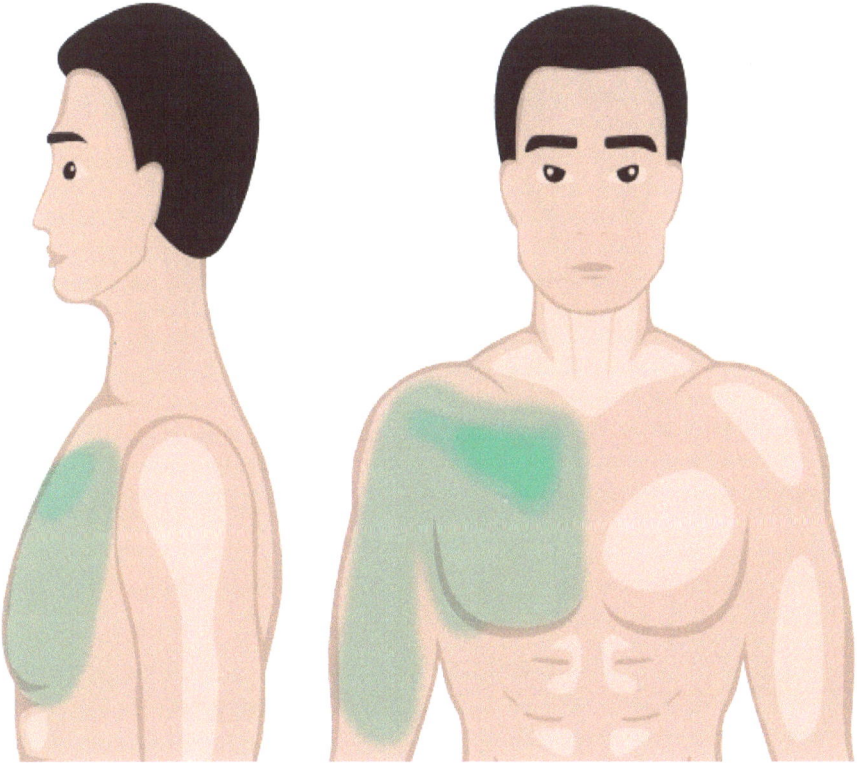

You can move the arm to have easier access to the muscle.

Pectoralis minor (continued)

ℹ️ Reason for the tensions: you will often find tensions when clients lean forward and/or have their arms in wrong postures.

Which area to target :

- The muscle can be neglected during a pectoralis massage if you do not take the necessary time to palpate and relax it.

Self-massage tools	Use
Ball	The ball can rapidly isolate and relax the muscle with direct pressure.
Exercises	You will have to be sure to isolate the muscle if you want to stretch it correctly. This type of stretch requires more attention to detail and precision to obtain the desired result.
Massage gun	The gun can release a muscle that's always tensed and help it relax. The ball head attachment is recommended.

Self-massage tools

Our muscles and the tools to relax them

Use the right tool for the right muscle with this table, but do not hesitate to explore them all.

Muscles	Ball	Foam roller	Exercises	Massage gun
Adductors		⬚		✓
Biceps	🎾		🧘	✓
Biceps brachialis	🎾		🧘	✓
Calf	🎾	⬚		✓
Clavicle	🎾			✓
Deltoid	🎾			✓
Elbow	🎾			✓
Finger extensor			🧘	✓
Finger flexor			🧘	✓

Our muscles and the tools to relax them (continued)

Muscles	Ball	Foam roller	Exercises	Massage gun
Foot	🎾			✓
Forearm	🎾		🧘	✓
Glutes	🎾	▯	🧘	✓
Hand	🎾			✓
Hamstring		▯	🧘	✓
Levator scapulae	🎾		🧘	
Neck	🎾			
Occiput	🎾			
Pectoralis major	🎾		🧘	✓
Pectoralis minor	🎾	▯	🧘	✓

Our muscles and the tools to relax them (continued)

Muscles	Ball	Foam roller	Exercises	Massage gun
Psoas			🧘	
Quadriceps		▯	🧘	✓
Quadriceps lateralis		▯	🧘	✓
Rhomboid	🎾			
Rotator cuff	🎾		🧘	✓
Spinalis		▯	🧘	
Subscapularis			🧘	
Tensor fasciae latae (TFL)	🎾			✓
Tibialis anterior	🎾			✓
Triceps	🎾		🧘	✓

Choosing
the right tool

Common tools for self-massaging

Massage ball

You can use the ball for spots that require precision and for your arms, forearms, and pectorals muscles.

Exercises

The exercises can be helpful for someone who seems really tense and has a hard time relaxing his/her muscles with the a self-massage.

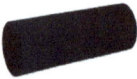

Foam roller

You can effectively use the roller for the largest muscles, such as the legs, the glutes, and the hamstrings. You can also use it to relax your back.

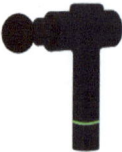

Massage gun

This tool is recommended when you feel your skin is tight, a sore muscle, or you feel your mobility is reduced. It is, however, unable to reach the deepest tensions.

Complete your collection

Also available in this collection

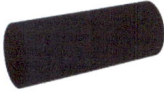

Foam roller

https://massoguide.com/u0jm

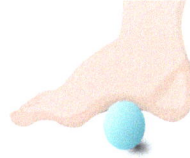

Massage ball

https://massoguide.com/i09r

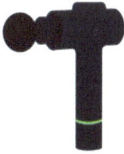

Massage gun

https://massoguide.com/qn8v

Exercises

https://massoguide.com/5e35

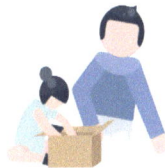

Bad postures

https://massoguide.com/i2yb

Specialized guides for massage therapists

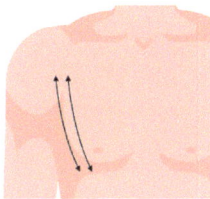

Techniques for good pressure:
Thinking differently

https://massoguide.com/4jax

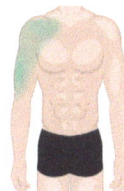

Massage techniques to relieve
muscle tension

https://massoguide.com/azoc

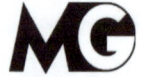

Find your tool

Use the opinions of massage exports on the different self-massage products available.

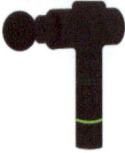

Massage gun

- Batteries
- Accessories

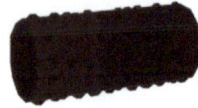

Foam roller

- Lengths
- Surfaces

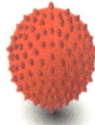

Massage ball

- Sizes
- Surfaces

Help us by sharing your feedback on this guide:

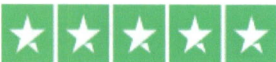

★★★★★

Please! Leave a testimonial

massoguide.com/bdi7

Share on
Facebook!

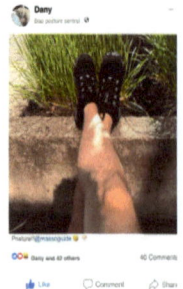